New Perspectives in Behavioral & Health Sciences

New Perspectives in Behavioral & Health Sciences is a series of high-quality, compact volumes focused on presenting interdisciplinary perspectives on key, developing, or new topics in Behavioral and Health Sciences. This SpringerBrief series will be of interest to a broad range of researchers and practitioners working in related fields of Behavioral and Health Sciences such as Psychology, Mental Health, Criminology, Public Health, and Social Work.

Suchismita Satapathy ·
Arturo Realyvásquez Vargas · Meghana Mishra

Mental and Occupational Stress Assessment of Pink Collar Workers

Springer

Suchismita Satapathy
School of Mechanical Engineering
KIIT University
Bhubaneswar, Odisha, India

Arturo Realyvásquez Vargas
Department of Industrial Engineering
Tecnológico Nacional de México
Tijuana, Baja California, Mexico

Meghana Mishra
Kalinga Institute of Industrial Technology
Bhubaneswar, Odisha, India

ISSN 2731-9296 ISSN 2731-930X (electronic)
New Perspectives in Behavioral & Health Sciences
ISBN 978-981-97-9597-0 ISBN 978-981-97-9598-7 (eBook)
https://doi.org/10.1007/978-981-97-9598-7

This Springer imprint is published by the registered company Springer Nature Singapore Pte Ltd.
The registered company address is: 152 Beach Road, #21-01/04 Gateway East, Singapore 189721, Singapore

Preface

This book includes seven chapters, which focus on the physical, psychological, and mental stress of pink-collar workers in different services such as hotels, nursery teaching, and care taking. A pink-collar worker is a person employed in a care-related profession or in an area that has traditionally been seen as the domain of women. Jobs in the beauty business, nursing, social work, education, teaching, secretarial work, upholstery, or child care are just a few examples. Although males may hold these positions as well, historically women have held the majority of them.Because gender barriers have continuously eroded in recent years, the distinction between employment that is geared towards men and women is becoming increasingly hazy. However, there is still gender segregation in many professions. This may be a result of institutional barriers, cultural norms, and social expectations that have a disproportionate impact on the representation of women in pink-collar positions. Although women still dominate the nursing profession, men have recently begun to enter the field. In other words, nursing has evolved into a good career option for people of any gender who want to work in medicine. Even before the phrase "pink-collar job" was created in 1970, teachers in grades K-12 were typically female. Teaching is a profession that benefits society, and students develop and learn via face-to-face encounters. The majority of teachers in kindergarten and preschool are still women (more than 97%).

Early childhood educators focus on the social and physical needs, as well as the learning and development of small children as these young minds want to explore the world, so proper care will enable the development of small children, not only to ensure they become physically fit but also mentally well and able to face the challenges of life.

A teacher's responsibility is to create a welcoming and secure atmosphere where young children can develop their social, physical, and adaptive skills as well as their early academic abilities (math, science, social studies, and reading skills). Pink-collar workers are engaged in their job for eight to ten hours a day, sacrificing family time. So, the time factor is a main stressor for these workers. To satisfy the financial requirements of the family, pink-collar workers have to spend their time working day and night. They have to face many difficulties such as emotional hardship (e.g. dealing with patients or clients), the workload, interpersonal conflicts, and job insecurity. So this book is an effort to study pink-collar workers' challenges and to suggest valid solutions to them.

Hence, in Chap. 1, a detailed discussion about the stress factors and occupational health and safety factors of pink-collar workers is provided and measures are suggested to reduce mental pressure in the work place. Chapter 2 provides a clear account of the mental health and occupational hazards of pink-collar workers by way of a literature review. Chapters 3 and 4 provide a pictorial representation of the physical health and cause of stressors of pink-collar workers in health care and of nursery teachers. Chapter 5 focuses on a design framework to mitigate the challenges of pink-collar workers in different services. Chapter 6 describes the physical and mental stress in hotel services. Chapter 7 concludes with recent statistics on pink-collar workers and their future.

Bhubaneswar, India — Suchismita Satapathy
Tijuana, Mexico — Arturo Realyvásquez Vargas
Bhubaneswar, India — Meghana Mishra

About This Book

This book is about the challenges of pink-collar workers and their mental and physical health. The authors will describe the physical work load involved and the mental health consequences of different kinds of work place. They will also design a framework to reduce the mental load of pink-collar workers. Lastly the contemporary status of pink-collar workers will be explored.

Contents

1 Introduction 1
1.1 Stress Factors for Pink-Collar Workers 1
1.2 Occupational Health of Pink-Collar Workers and Its Effect on the Economic, Social, Cultural, and Technical Conditions of an Emerging Economy 2
1.3 Measures to Reduce Stress for Pink-Collar Workers 2
1.4 Conclusion 3

2 Review of Mental Health and Work Place Hazards 5
2.1 Literature Review of Work Place Hazards and Stressors for Pink-Collar Workers 5
2.2 Literature Review on Safety and Sustainability Measures for Pink-Collar Workers 6
2.3 Conclusion 7
References 7

3 Assessment of Stressors and Risk Factors of Nurses Engaged in Healthcare Services 11
3.1 Introduction 11
3.2 Research Methodology 12
3.3 Results and Discussion 13
3.4 Conclusion 16
References 17

4 Evaluation of Risks and Mental Health for Nursery Staff, School Teachers, and Child Care Workers 19
4.1 Introduction 19
4.2 Research Methodology 20
4.3 Results and Discussion 20
4.4 Conclusion 23
References 23

5 Designing a Framework to Reduce the Mental Work Load and Improve the Mental Health of Workers Engaged in Pink-Collar Jobs 25
5.1 Introduction 25
5.2 Research Methodology 25
5.3 Results and Discussion 26
5.4 Conclusion 29
References 29

6 Exploring the Physical and Mental Pressure of Workers in Hotel Services 31
6.1 Introduction 31
6.2 Research Methodology 32
6.3 Results and Discussion 33
6.4 Conclusion 37
References 37

7 Conclusion and Study of the Changing Scenario of the Pink-Collar-Worker Industry 39
7.1 Introduction 39
7.2 Study of the Changing Scenario of the Pink-Collar Industry 39
7.3 Methodology 40
7.4 Results and Discussion 41
7.4.1 Conclusion and Future Scope 44

Index 45

About the Authors

Suchismita Satapathy is an associate professor in the School of Mechanical Sciences, KIIT University, Bhubaneswar, India. She has published more than 130 articles in national and international journals and conferences. She has also published many books and e-books for academic and research purposes. Her areas of interest include production operation management, operation research, acoustics, sustainability, and supply chain management. She has filed three Indian patents, two of which have been published. She has more than 15 years of teaching and research experience. She has supervised many Ph.D. (three completed, three ongoing), M.Tech. (20), and B.Tech. (49) students. She has published books such as *Production Operation Management* (Stadium Press) and *MCDM Methods for Waste Management* (CRC Press), *Innovation, Technology, and Knowledge Management* (Springer), *Soft Computing and Optimization Techniques for Sustainable Agriculture* (De Gruyter), and *The PDCA Cycle for Industrial Improvement, Applied Case Studies* (Springer); many of her projects are ongoing.
Scopus Author ID: 55085975400

Arturo Realyvásquez Vargas is a full-time professor at the Department of Industrial Engineering at Tecnológico Nacional de Mexico/Instituto Tecnológico de Tijuana in Mexico. He received a master's degree in Industrial Engineering and a Ph.D. in Engineering Sciences from the Autonomous University of Ciudad Juarez in Mexico. Currently, he is studying a Ph.D. in Innovation in Product Engineering and Industrial Process at the University of La Rioja (Spain). In addition, his main research areas are related to the optimization of industrial processes, lean manufacturing, and ergonomics. He is an active member of the Society of Ergonomists of Mexico Civil Association (Sociedad de Ergonomistas de México, SEMAC) and the Network of Optimization of Industrial Processes (Red de Optimización de Procesos Industriales, ROPRIN). Currently, he is a National Researcher recognized by the National Council of Science & Technology of Mexico (CONACYT) at level I. He is also an author/coauthor of 12 papers published in journals indexed in the Journal Citation Reports. He has attended international conferences and congresses in Mexico and the United States of America.
Scopus Author ID: 56167726800.

Meghana Mishra is a research scholar in the School of Commerce at KIIT University, Bhubaneswar, India. She has published 10 articles in national and international journals as well as book chapters. Her areas of interest include production operation management, the economic study of the agrisector, sustainability, business process reengineering, and ergonomics.
Scopus Author ID: 58131312900

Abbreviations

AI	Artificial intelligence
CCTV	Closed-circuit television
DASS	Depression anxiety stress scale
FA	Factor analysis
HoQ	House of quality
ILO	International labour organisation
IoT	Internet of Things
MCDM	Multi-criteria decision-making
MSDs	Musculoskeletal disorders
OHS	Occupational health and safety
OSHA	Occupational safety and health administration
PSS	Perceived stress scale
QFD	Quality function deployment
WASPAS	Weighted aggregate sum and product assessment

List of Figures

Fig. 3.1 Selection of nurses country-wise 13
Fig. 5.1 Number of selected workers 27
Fig. 5.2 Number of selected workers gender-wise 27
Fig. 5.3 House of quality 29
Fig. 6.1 Selected number of workers country-wise 32
Fig. 6.2 ISM model 36
Fig. 6.3 MICMAC analysis 36
Fig. 7.1 Residual plot 42

List of Tables

Table 3.1	Questionnaire	12
Table 3.2	Selection of nurses by age and work experience	13
Table 3.3	Factor analysis	14
Table 3.4	Decision matrix	14
Table 3.5	Normalized matrix	15
Table 3.6	Ranking	15
Table 3.7	Cause of risk factors in nursing jobs	16
Table 4.1	Risk factors in child care jobs	20
Table 4.2	Factor analysis	21
Table 4.3	Selected nursery teachers' percentage score	21
Table 4.4	PSS scale	22
Table 4.5	PSS scores for teachers (pink-collar employees)	23
Table 5.1	Customer requirements/challenges for pink-collar workers	26
Table 5.2	Requirements for mitigating challenges	26
Table 5.3	Designed House of Quality	28
Table 6.1	Questionnaire	32
Table 6.2	Types of workers	33
Table 6.3	Factor analysis	33
Table 6.4	Self structural interactive matrix	33
Table 6.5	Initial reachability matrix	34
Table 6.6	Final reachability matrix with transitivity relationship	34
Table 6.7	Iteration 1	34
Table 6.8	Iteration 2	35
Table 6.9	Iteration 3	35
Table 6.10	Iteration 4	35
Table 6.11	MIC MAC analysis	35
Table 7.1	Opinions on the changes in the pink-collar industry	41
Table 7.2	Pink-collar workers who report a positive response (%)	41
Table 7.3	Criteria for pink-collar workers	43
Table 7.4	Alternatives	43
Table 7.5	Decision matrix criteria	43

Table 7.6 Normalized values 43
Table 7.7 Positive and negative ideal solutions 44
Table 7.8 Ranking 44

Chapter 1
Introduction

1.1 Stress Factors for Pink-Collar Workers

Those who work in service-oriented positions that are typically associated with women are known as pink-collar workers. These positions frequently place a strong emphasis on caring and interpersonal skills. Although the phrase was first used in the late 1970s, its definition has now expanded to encompass any career that values traits that are often associated with women.

Pink-collar jobs are divided into two types:

- Care oriented;
- Administrative.

Nursing, health care, child care, nursery school teachers, hotel services, and beauty industries are termed care-oriented jobs. Waiters, retail sales clerks and the like are termed administrative jobs. Care-oriented jobs also vary in nature. But the nature of all such jobs is long working hours and repetitive in nature.

Pink-collar jobs are more service-oriented job and require a lot of physical as well as emotional labor. They need a lot of patience and emotional intelligence to handle small children, angry and aggressive customers, and senior citizens. The low wage rate and discrimination makes these workers stressed, as they face sexual harassment, mental pressure, musculoskeletal disorders, and are also unable to balance their family life.

S. Satapathy et al., *Mental and Occupational Stress Assessment of Pink Collar Workers*, New Perspectives in Behavioral & Health Sciences,
https://doi.org/10.1007/978-981-97-9598-7_1

1.2 Occupational Health of Pink-Collar Workers and Its Effect on the Economic, Social, Cultural, and Technical Conditions of an Emerging Economy

Pink-collar jobs are meant to provide physical and mental care for small children and elderly people, patients, and so on. As these workers are frequently providing care for others, emotional hardship, stress, and burnout can have a negative impact on an employee's health. These positions frequently pay less and call for employees to regulate their emotions as well as to show empathy and support for others. Under this huge pressure the occupational risks of pink-collar workers are very high. They may experience stress, anxiety, and aggression during their work, which will have an effect on their mental and physical health. These workers' occupational health has a big impact on their personal life and also on the social, cultural, technological, and economic aspects of emerging countries as follows.

- Social Impact: If these pink-collar workers are unwell, physically sick, or mentally unwell, they will not able to take care of others' health. Hence work performance will decrease and the quality of care will also be affected. Due to the poor occupational health female participation or involvement may be limited in pink-collar jobs, which will have an effect on their economic freedom.
- Cultural Impact: Poor occupational health may prohibit the participation of female workers and change the culture as they face problems in making their work and family life balance, resulting in a negative mentality towards pink-collar jobs and the female community not participating.
- Technological Impact: Providing work place safety and an ergonomically comfortable work place, by implementing advanced technology, will cause many to become pink-collar workers and perform their duties comfortably. Proper training will result in such workers being more skilled and not facing any problems.
- Economic Impact: Pink-collar jobs create income inequality, which will deflect people from working and negatively impact the economy of developing countries. Due to poor occupational health, absenteeism will increase and productivity will reduce.

1.3 Measures to Reduce Stress for Pink-Collar Workers

Pink-collar workers are very important for society. Hence some measures must be taken to reduce the mental and physical stress of these workers:

- In the work place, sufficient workers must be present to provide support;
- Flexible working hours and a digital work culture with a remote work system may reduce stress;
- Stress management training programs and career counseling may help in making pink-collar workers more happy in the work place;

- Redistribution of tasks and providing work allowances and breaks will help in the reduction of mental stress;
- Providing yoga, gym and meditation facilities in the work place may help workers to be more healthy physically and mentally;
- An ergonomic work place, fair wages, flexibility, and freedom to speak out may help pink-collar workers to love their work place and their sense of belonging will increase;
- With a recognition, award, and appreciation system, pink-collar workers will increase their sense of belonging.

1.4 Conclusion

Pink-collar employment concerns jobs where women predominate, although nowadays males are also doing the same type of job. Although there has been improvement in the area of gender equality, the sad truth is that some workplaces or areas still have the percentage of female participation at a maximum. In the twenty-first century, these jobs are still underappreciated and paid less than those held by males.

When you combine this with the reality that women sometimes perform an unpaid "second shift" at home, it becomes clear why the gender parity deck is still loaded against women despite their advancements. Not only are they unpaid, their job remains unrecognized and taken for granted. These women suffer a lot to balance their work life and family life. In the work place they give their best, but are still not appreciated like men. With a nominal wage rate, such a work burden, without appreciation, and without support these pink-collar workers work day and night. Sometimes they suffer violence, sexual harassment, and so on. And they don't get social respect like their male partners.

As health care workers in hospitals, with patients, there may be contact with biological hazards or risks due to pathogens or blood infections. Night duties, rotating shifts, and taking care of patients' physical and mental health make them fatigued and mentally sick. As carers, these workers have to attend to small children and senior/old persons. So they became mentally and physically affected by ergonomic hazards. Even in hospitality, dealing with a variety of customers/clients and fulfilling their demands makes this a very challenging job. These workers suffer with physical pain and mental hazards in performing these responsibilities in the work place. Specific hours of work, standard wage rates, consistent regulations, and support from higher management may help them to mitigate these challenges and make the work place comfortable.

Chapter 2
Review of Mental Health and Work Place Hazards

2.1 Literature Review of Work Place Hazards and Stressors for Pink-Collar Workers

Lips-Wiersma et al. (2016) compared pink-collar workers with white collar workers. Sullivan and Hodson (2002) have described pink-collar jobs as service based jobs. Casey (2012) has classified pink-collar jobs as including office assistant jobs, hotel services, nursery school teachers, and healthcare services. Briggs (2005) has mapped the percentages of pink-collar workers by Environmental Systems Research Institute ArcGIS 10. Lips-Wiersma et al. (2016) made a comparison between white, pink, and blue-collar workers by observing the frequency of jobs. The US Department of Labor—Bureau of Labor statistics (2006) has termed pink-collar workers as personal service oriented workers. Barnes et al. (2021) explained that due to the lower number of pink-collar workers they are not calculated in economic budgets. Chun et al. (2020) studied depression in pink-collar workers due to emotional hardship. Wang and Gorenstein (2014) conducted a study on depression in the work place. Evans-Lacko and Knapp (2016) have shown that absenteeism in the work place is due to depression. Henderson et al. (2014) found that nowadays many people are sick due to depression in the work place. Härmä et al. (2006), Zapf et al. (1999), and Lee (2015) found that the main cause of depression among pink-collar workers is the work place environment. Clark (2013) showed that as growth in the manufacturing sector moved to the service sector, so pink-collar jobs gained more prominence. Yun et al. (2019) have shown that pink-collar workers have to follow companies' rules that involve emotional hardship. Zapf (2002) has shown that emotional hardship has both a positive and negative impact on the health of pink-collar workers. Seo et al. (2018) have shown that there has been less research conducted on health and safety information for pink-collar workers.

S. Satapathy et al., *Mental and Occupational Stress Assessment of Pink Collar Workers*, New Perspectives in Behavioral & Health Sciences,
https://doi.org/10.1007/978-981-97-9598-7_2

2.2 Literature Review on Safety and Sustainability Measures for Pink-Collar Workers

The Manusmriti's publication raised concerns about women's status in society, and the caste system that characterized Vedic culture during that time further reinforced a narrow, patriarchal viewpoint through epics and scholarly discourse (Mohapatra 2015).

In India, the term "pink-colorization" describes the tendency of a large proportion of women working in low-paying, historically female-dominated fields. The clustering of women in areas including education, healthcare, and services—where they frequently perform care giving, support, or regular administrative duties—defines this phenomenon. Social conceptions of gender roles are a major factor in the pink-colorization of the workforce. Women are frequently led by deeply ingrained cultural norms toward professions that are viewed as socially acceptable or conventionally feminine. The perception that teaching, nursing, and administrative positions are suited for women sometimes results in a concentration of female employees in these sectors. The World Bank (2020) notes that 88.06% of females in India prefer a nursing job.

Robyn et al. (2000) developed an effective measuring tool for the safety climate of hospitals. Rogers and Travers (1991), McAbee et al. (1993), Sepkowitz (1996), and Moore and Kaczmarek (1990) have discussed the biological, physical, chemical, and ergonomic hazards that are a risk for workers in the hospitality sector. DiBenedetto (1995), Grant (1993), and Zhang et al. (2021) have reported that hospital workers' and nurses' weak health is caused by rotating shifts, heavy work loads, a lack of autonomy, and poor supervision. Zohar (1980) has noted that workers' perception of the work place is very important when assessing whether it is safe or unsafe. Finn et al. (2024) have pointed out that long-term stress can be mitigated by strong institutional support.

As indicated by Chandra et al. (2013), Coiera and Hovenga (2007), Berwick and Hackbarth (2012), Barjis et al. (2013), and Arce-Corrales et al. (2014), sustainability acts like a guard to protect the natural environment, human health, and the planet. It also takes care of new innovations. Coiera and Hovenga (2007) have shown that the negative environmental effects of healthcare can be minimized with the help of sustainability, which also provides easy access of service, stability, and low cost. Klangsin and Harding (1998) have shown that sustainability can reduce biohazard pollution and make the environment safe, resulting in hospital staff being kept safe from infection.

To create a more sustainable future for people and the environment, sustainable practices that lessen their negative effects on the environment, preserve natural resources, and safeguard the health and safety of employees are essential. However, policies for safety and sustainability in the work place are especially important in sectors of the economy that have a large environmental impact or present serious occupational hazards.

2.3 Conclusion

Companies can foster a health-focused culture that improves employee well-being and job satisfaction in order to support them with mental health issues. In addition to being a basic human right, safe and healthy work environments can reduce stress and disputes at work and enhance employee retention, output, and performance. On the other hand, a lack of supportive systems and efficient procedures at work, particularly for those with mental health issues, can negatively impact an individual's capacity to enjoy and perform their job; it can also erode people's confidence in their abilities.

Social risks at work is also key to preventing mental health disorders. Employers are advised by the WHO to accomplish this by putting in place organizational interventions that specifically address the surroundings and working conditions. Organizational interventions evaluate workplace risks to mental health and then take steps to reduce, eliminate, or change those risks. Organizational interventions can take the form of introducing frameworks to address workplace violence and harassment or offering flexible work schedules.

References

Arce-Corrales, M. E., Gomez-Alvarez, A., & Alvarez-Chavez, C. R. (2014). Chemical substances sources characterization in support of the health sector's sustainability and quality in Sonora, Mexico. Journal of Cleaner Production, 64, 457–463.

Barjis, J., Kolfschoten, G., & Maritz, J. (2013). A sustainable and affordable support system for rural healthcare delivery. Decision Support Systems, 56, 223–233.

Barnes TD, Beall VD, Holman MR. Pink-collar representation and budgetary outcomes in US states. Legislative Studies Quarterly. 2021 Feb;46(1):119–54.

Basu S, Ratcliffe G, Green M. Health and pink-collar work. Occupational Medicine. 2015 Oct 1;65(7):529–34.

Berwick, D. M., & Hackbarth, A. D. (2012). Eliminating waste in US health care. Jama, 307(14), 1513–1516.

Briggs D. The role of GIS: coping with space (and time) in air pollution exposure assessment. Journal of Toxicology and Environmental Health, Part A. 2005 Jul 1;68(13–14):1243–61.

Casey C. The changing contexts of work. In Understanding learning at work 2012 Oct 12 (pp. 15–28). Routledge.

Chandra, H., Rinkoo, A. V., Verma, J. K., Kapoor, R., & Sharma, R. (2013). Supply chain management with cost containment & financial sustainability in a tertiary care hospital. Journal of Health & Human Services Administration, Summer, 36(1), 3–23.

Chun HR, Cho I, Choi Y, Cho SI. Effects of emotional labor factors and working environment on the risk of depression in pink-collar workers. International journal of environmental research and public health. 2020 Jul;17(14):5208.

Clark D. *Urban. Decline (Routledge Revivals)* Routledge; New York, NY, USA: 2013.

Coiera, E., &Hovenga, E. J. S. (2007). Building a sustainable health system. Yearbook of Medical Informatics, 46, 11–18.

DiBenedetto DV. Occupational hazards of the health care industry: protecting health care workers. AAOHN Journal. 1995 Mar;43(3):131–7.

Evans-Lacko S., Knapp M. Global patterns of workplace productivity for people with depression: Absenteeism and presenteeism costs across eight diverse countries. *Soc. Psychiatry Psychiatr. Epidemiol.* 2016;**51**:1525–1537. https://doi.org/10.1007/s00127-016-1278-4

Finn M, Walsh A, Rafter N, Mellon L, Chong HY, Naji A, O'Brien N, Williams DJ, McCarthy SE. Effect of interventions to improve safety culture on healthcare workers in hospital settings: a systematic review of the international literature. BMJ Open Quality. 2024 May 1;13(2):e002506.

Grant PS. Manage nurse stress and increase potential at the bedside. Nursing Administration Quarterly. 1993 Oct 1;18(1):16–22.

Härmä M., Kompier M.A.J., Vahtera J. Work-related stress and health—risks, mechanisms and countermeasures. *Scand. J. Work Health.* 2006;**32**:413–419. https://doi.org/10.5271/sjweh.1047

Henderson M., Madan I., Hotopf M. *Work and Mental Health in the UK.* British Medical Journal Publishing Group; London, UK: 2014.

Klangsin, P., & Harding, A. K. (1998). Medical waste treatment and disposal methods used by hospitals in Oregon, Washington, and Idaho. Journal of the Air & Waste Management Association, 48(6), 516–526.

Lee G. Korean emotional laborers' job stressors and relievers: Focus on work conditions and emotional labor properties. *Saf. Health Work.* 2015;**6**:338–344.

Lips-Wiersma M, Wright S, Dik B. Meaningful work: differences among blue-, pink-, and white-collar occupations. Career Develop Int 21(5):534–51.

McAbee RR, Gallucci BJ, Checkoway H. Adverse reproductive outcomes and occupational exposures among nurses: an investigation of multiple hazardous exposures. AAOHN Journal. 1993 Mar;41(3):110–9.

Mohapatra, H. (2015). Status of Women in Indian Society. Quest Journals Journal of Research in Humanities and Social Science, 3(6), 2321–9467. www.questjournals.org

Moore Jr RM, Kaczmarek RG. Occupational hazards to health care workers: diverse, ill-defined, and not fully appreciated. American Journal of Infection Control. 1990 Oct 1;18(5):316–27.

Rogers B, Travers P. Overview of work-related hazards in nursing: Health and safety issues. Heart & lung: the journal of critical care. 1991 Sep 1;20(5 Pt 1):486–97.

S. Department of Labor – Bureau of Labor Statistics (24 May 2006). "Occupational Employment and Wages – Waiters and Waitresses". US Department of Labor. Retrieved 31 December 2006.

Seo J.I., Shin G.S., Kim M.G., Min Y.S. Relationship between occupational injuries and the provision of safety and health information: Data from the 4th Korean working conditions survey. *Ann. Occup. Environ. Med.* 2018;**30**:36.

Sepkowitz KA. Occupationally acquired infections in health care workers: part I. Annals of internal medicine. 1996 Nov 15;125(10):826–34.

Sullivan TA, Hodson R. The social organization of work. Wadsworth Publishing Company; 2002.

Wang Y.-P., Gorenstein C. Attitude and impact of perceived depression in the workplace. *Int. J. Environ. Res. Public Health.* 2014;**11**:6021–6036.

Yun S., Lim S.S., Kim J., Kim Y.K., Won J.U., Yoon J.H. The role of customer service manual on workplace emotional burden in nationwide cross sectional study. *Ann. Occup. Environ. Med.* 2019;**31**:5. https://doi.org/10.1186/s40557-019-0285-9

Zapf D., Vogt C., Seifert C., Mertini H., Isic A. Emotion Work as a Source of Stress: The Concept and Development of an Instrument. *Eur. J. Work Organ. Psychol.* 1999;**8**:371–400. https://doi.org/10.1080/135943299398230

Zapf D. Emotion work and psychological well-being: A review of the literature and some conceptual considerations. *Hum. Resour. Manag. Rev.* 2002;**12**:237–268. https://doi.org/10.1016/S1053-4822(02)00048-7

Zhang M, Murphy B, Cabanilla A, Yidi C. Physical relaxation for occupational stress in healthcare workers: A systematic review and network meta-analysis of randomized controlled trials. Journal of occupational health. 2021 Jan;63(1):e12243.

Zohar D. Safety climate in industrial organizations: theoretical and applied implications. Journal of applied psychology. 1980 Feb;65(1):96.

Chapter 3
Assessment of Stressors and Risk Factors of Nurses Engaged in Healthcare Services

3.1 Introduction

Workplace hazards exist for most field workers, and often, in many professional spaces and official jobs (without field work), a worker is employed for eight to ten hours, including shifts both in day time and night time. These jobs are very hectic and employees suffer from many types of health and mental disorders. They also face mental stress and discomfort when sleeping. Nurses are included in the pink-collar workers category as they take care of patients, perform administrative jobs, and so on. Pink-collar work is usually considered to be done by females. Nurses have to take care of patients, participate in surgery/operations, take care of medicines, and perform routine check-ups. Hence, they have great responsibilities and undertake a physical work load in performing their duties. Despite their heavy work load, their pay package is much less than that of other professions. Their job has no growth or promotion in future. Pink-collar workers, including nurses, are usually under-valued compared to other jobs. They also face many types of challenges and risks in the work place. Ngowi et al. (2001) discussed toxicity and its effects on the physical and mental health of coffee workers in Tanzania. Arvidsson et al. (2012) discussed the health and mental strain of metal-cutting workers. Basu et al. (2015) assessed the health outcome of both pink and blue-collar workers. Chun et al. (2020) performed a comparison between male and female pink-collar workers using logistic regression analysis. Bernhagen and Gravett (2017) have discussed about the entry of women shows best response then men in education sector.

During patient care, nurses face a high risk of contamination. They also have to do night duties regularly, so they face challenges in their personal and family lives. Abdoh et al. (2021) explored the stressors of the nurses of Saudi Arabia using the DASS scale. Zavadskas et al. (2012) did the same using the WASPAS method.

S. Satapathy et al., *Mental and Occupational Stress Assessment of Pink Collar Workers*, New Perspectives in Behavioral & Health Sciences,
https://doi.org/10.1007/978-981-97-9598-7_3

3.2 Research Methodology

Although there have been many changes to the nursing profession, many of these pink-collar workers still have to face many challenges. So following our extensive literature review we designed a questionnaire based on the challenges and risk factors of nurses at their work place and in their profession. This was then distributed among 389 nurses in developing countries including India, Nigeria, Mexico, Bangladesh, and Nepal. Their responses were categorized according to the Likert scale (where 1 = disagree; 2 = no opinion; 3 = agree). Further statistical and WASPAS (weighted aggregated sum product assessment) method (like Marcos) analysis was implemented to prioritize stressors and risk factors. Table 3.1 shows the questionnaire. Figure 3.1 shows the selection of nurses country-wise. Table 3.2 shows the selected nurses on the basis of age and work experience, and reveals that nurses in the age band 35–45 had the most work experience of 12–15 years. From Fig. 3.1 it is clear that most nurses were selected from India and Mexico. Factor analysis was then conducted, followed by the WASPAS MCDM method.

Table 3.1 Questionnaire

	Questionnaire	1	2	3
1	Nurse handles many types of patients suffering from different diseases			
2	They suffer high work pressure due to overload at work			
3	They have to deal with pain, life, and death			
4	They have career related worries			
5	They have to cope with and adopt various technologies			
6	Coworkers can be competitive			
7	They struggle and fight with administration and coworkers			
8	Behavior of doctors			
9	Sleeplessness during day and night shifts			
10	Lack of family time			
11	Job insecurity			
12	Struggling with work pressure due to lack of staff			
13	Lack of facilities and resources			
14	Emotionally attached to patients but feeling helpless			
15	No flexibility in working hours			
16	Unable to balance family time and work time			
17	Wage rate is low			
18	Temporary position			
19	Risk of infection			
20	Lack of management support			

Table 3.2 Selection of nurses by age and work experience

Age	Experience (years)	No. of nurses
18–25	0–5	42
25–35	8–12	73
35–45	12–15	122
45–55	20–25	118
55–65	30–40	34

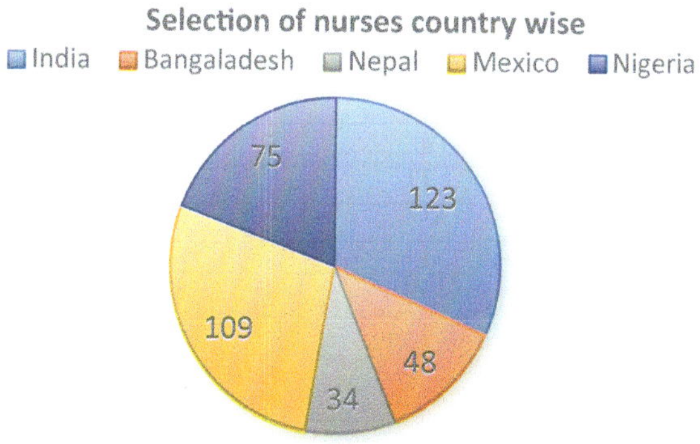

Fig. 3.1 Selection of nurses country-wise

3.3 Results and Discussion

Statistical analysis of the data was done to find the most important stressors. In the first phase, factor analysis was conducted using Minitab 17 for 20 items under 7 constructs, namely Workload and Time Pressure, Emotional and Psychological Stress, Interpersonal Relationships, Organizational and Environmental Factors, Physical Demands, and Job Insecurity and Personal Life Stressors. Items below the accepted Cronbach's value of 0.5 were not considered (see Table 3.3).

To find the most important stressors for nursing pink-collar workers, the WASPAS method was used to rank alternatives. This is a more precise method than other MCDM methods.

The steps of the WASPAS method are:

- Develop decision matrix;
- Normalize decision matrix;
- Find Q1 and Q2, as weighted summation and weighted production;
- Then find total Q = 0.5 * Q1 + 0.5 * Q2;
- Then find ranking.

The WASPAS method was implemented to prioritize stress factors. Tables 3.4, 3.5 and 3.6 show ranking by this method.

From Table 3.6, which shows ranking by the WASPAS method, it is clear that nurses feel stressed when they have major problems coping with and adopting to

Table 3.3 Factor analysis

	Item	F1	F2	F3	F4	F5	F6	F7
Workload and time pressure	2 9 15	0.501 0.532 0.528						
Emotional and psychological stress	3 14		0.603 0.552					
Interpersonal relationships	6 7 8			0.535 0.509 0.511				
Physical demands	18 19				0.562 0.618			
Job security	4 11 17					0.602 0.583 0.613		
Organizational and environmental factor	13 20						0.519 0.701	
Personal life stressors	1 10							0.639 0.726

Table 3.4 Decision matrix

Stressors	Private hospitals	Government hospitals	Dispensaries
1	3.4	4.23	3.432
2	2.3	3.067	2.698
3	2.93	3.28	4.12
4	3.6	4.07	3.78
5	3.5	4.63	3.84
6	4.5	3.29	2.94
7	3.056	3.11	4.12
8	4.12	4.29	2.76
9	3.05	3.17	4.53
10	3.27	2.876	4.12
11	4.12	4.11	3.207
12	3.98	2.46	3.65
13	4.887	3.067	4.07
14	4.13	4.35	2.05
15	3.05	3.76	3.34
16	3.27	3.03	3.14
17	2.19	2.95	2.875

Table 3.5 Normalized matrix

Stressors	Private hospitals	Government hospitals	Dispensaries
1	0.695723348	0.913606911	0.757615894
2	0.470636382	0.662419006	0.595584989
3	0.599549826	0.708423326	0.909492274
4	0.73664825	0.879049676	0.834437086
5	0.716185799	1	0.847682119
6	0.920810313	0.710583153	0.649006623
7	0.625332515	0.671706263	0.909492274
8	0.843052998	0.926565875	0.609271523
9	0.624104768	0.684665227	1
10	0.669122161	0.621166307	0.909492274
11	0.843052998	0.887688985	0.70794702
12	0.814405566	0.531317495	0.805739514
13	1	0.662419006	0.898454746
14	0.845099243	0.939524838	0.452538631
15	0.624104768	0.812095032	0.737306843
16	0.669122161	0.654427646	0.693156733
17	0.448127686	0.637149028	0.634657837

Table 3.6 Ranking

Stressors	Q1	Q2	Q	Rank
1	0.781092231	0.785729141	0.783410686	6th
2	0.570451325	0.573708743	0.572080034	16th
3	0.731763591	0.730605032	0.731184311	9th
4	0.808544554	0.816169138	0.812356846	3rd
5	0.846076413	0.8481553	0.847115856	Ist
6	0.752532029	0.753791593	0.753161811	8th
7	0.728155247	0.727929818	0.728042533	10th
8	0.785033831	0.782688367	0.783861099	5th
9	0.761894098	0.755340558	0.758617328	7th
10	0.725927645	0.725402529	0.725665087	14th
11	0.804767371	0.810883445	0.807825408	4th
12	0.70998265	0.706298915	0.708140782	12th
13	0.845088338	0.84261186	0.843850099	2nd
14	0.738263695	0.713354886	0.725809291	11th
15	0.717257192	0.722651926	0.719954559	13th
16	0.665513158	0.674722984	0.670118071	15th
17	0.567578402	0.56911523	0.568346816	17th

Table 3.7 Cause of risk factors in nursing jobs

	Questionnaire	1	0	Percentage
1	Young nurses faces more stress due to lack of experience			63.89
2	Female nurses may face work related stresses due to gender related roles and expectations			48.5
3	Rural area nurses may face problems due to lack of facilities			53.07
4	Nurses face more stress in emergency rooms			69.45
5	Nurses working in pediatric units are more stressed than in other departments			78.43
6	Lack of social or professional support increases stress			49.02

various technologies, which is ranked first. Lack of facilities and resources is the second highest cause of stress among pink-collar workers, and carrier related worries ranked third. Hence care must be taken to reduce or mitigate these stressors by proper training and educating nurses as to how to handle various and new technologies. By providing the requisite medical facilities and resources, the job of pink-collar workers will become easy.

Nurses have to face many risk factors in their profession. To assess their perception of these, the nurses were asked to answer with yes = 1 or no = 0 in their answers to the questionnaire shown in Table 3.7. This shows the cause of risk factors in nursing jobs; 69.45% of nurses are agreed that working in a pediatric unit is more stressful than in other departments, and 69.45% are agreed that nurses face more stress in emergency rooms.

3.4 Conclusion

We know that the impacts of stress have a negative effect on the mental health of a person and causes diseases like anxiety, depression, and exhaustion. Work place stress can cause musculoskeletal disorders and cardiovascular issues. This sickness will increase absenteeism in the work place and decrease productivity, job performance, and so on. Hence, the work policy for nurses must be taken care of properly. By including proper work allowance, wages, and rotation of work and shifts, the work life and family life of nurses can be balanced. Then, the nursing/healthcare profession might gain popularity.

References

Abdoh, D. S., Shahin, M. A., Ali, A. K., Alhejaili, S. M., Kiram, O. M., & Al-Dubai, S. A. R. (2021). Prevalence and associated factors of stress among primary health care nurses in Saudi Arabia, a multi-center study. *Journal of Family Medicine and Primary Care, 10*(7), 2692–2696.

Arvidsson I, Balogh I, Hansson GÅ, Ohlsson K, Åkesson I, Nordander C. Rationalization in meat cutting–consequences on physical workload. Applied Ergonomics. 2012 Nov 1;43(6):1026–32.

Basu S, Ratcliffe G, Green M. Health and pink-collar work. Occupational Medicine. 2015 Oct 1;65(7):529–34.

Bernhagen L, Gravett E. Educational development as pink collar labor: Implications and recommendations. To Improve the Academy. 2017 Jan;36(1):9–19.

Chun HR, Cho I, Choi Y, Cho SI. Effects of emotional labor factors and working environment on the risk of depression in pink-collar workers. International journal of environmental research and public health. 2020 Jul;17(14):5208.

Ngowi AV, Maeda DN, Partanen TJ, Sanga MP, Mbise G. Acute health effects of organophosphorus pesticides on Tanzanian small-scale coffee growers. Journal of Exposure Science & Environmental Epidemiology. 2001 Sep;11(4):335–9.

Zavadskas EK, Antuchevičienė J, Šaparauskas J, Turskis Z. MCDM methods WASPAS and MULTIMOORA: Verification of robustness of methods when assessing alternative solutions.

Chapter 4
Evaluation of Risks and Mental Health for Nursery Staff, School Teachers, and Child Care Workers

4.1 Introduction

Nursery school teachers and child care workers are employed day and night and need a lot of patience to take care of small children and sometimes infants. The number of children is sometimes large compared to carers and small infants display different states of mind like aggression, crying, or being playful. The energy level of small children is also very high. They need a lot of attention and care. As they learn by observing the behavior of their surrounding elders, teachers and carers need to exercise much precaution when teaching. As well as being in a playful mood children are also attention seekers. To gain attention or sometimes to explore, small nursery children might play with dangerous tools, fire, water, and so on. So these teachers have to observe them the whole day and also try to help them learn through various activities. To get them to engage teachers not only have to brain storm but also to make a lot of physical effort for them. The small child learns many lessons from the carer in absence of the parents. Hence the physical and mental well being of these carers and teachers is very important as their wellness also impacts on young minds, who are the future of society. So it is very crucial to evaluate the risks and mental health of nursery school teachers and child care workers. It is also clear that pressure due to the type of work they perform makes them stressed and has a direct effect on their mental well being and overall job performance. Čecho et al. (2019) explored the psychological stress of Kindergarten teachers. Fináncz et al. (2020) explored the relation between depression and work pressure. Faulkner et al. (2016) explained the main cause of mental stress as due to occupational stress among Kindergarten teachers of central Texas.

Although many researchers have investigated occupational stress and mental wellness, more research is required. Hence in this chapter the risks for and the mental health of nursery teachers are evaluated.

S. Satapathy et al., *Mental and Occupational Stress Assessment of Pink Collar Workers*, New Perspectives in Behavioral & Health Sciences,
https://doi.org/10.1007/978-981-97-9598-7_4

4.2 Research Methodology

To evaluate mental well being and the risks of child care and nursery teachers, an extensive literature review was conducted and a standard questionnaire designed. The survey was conducted for 420 nurses, school teachers and care takers of countries like India, Nepal,Bangaladesh, Nigeria. The survey was done using yes = 1 and no = 0 type questions. Then the mental risks for workers were evaluated after conducting factor analysis. To measure the mental risks for teachers, a perceived stress scale was employed (see Table 4.1).

4.3 Results and Discussion

The collected data were further analyzed using the factor analysis method. The 11 questions were distributed under 4 factors (i.e. physical stress, psychological stress, occupational stress, and work–life balance). Among 13 questions, 11 questions/items falling under 4 dimensions have a Cronbach's alpha value of more than 0.5; these were selected and the rest discarded (see Table 4.2).

From Table 4.3 it is clear that work load is high in educating and for caring has the highest score (87.45%), and the lowest score is for unsafe play areas or lack of sanitation.

To measure mental stress, a PSS scale was used.

Table 4.1 Risk factors in child care jobs

	Questionnaire	Yes = 1	No = 0	
1	Work load is high educating and for caring			
2	Exhausted emotionally			
3	Challenges in adjusting to the varying behavior of children			
4	Heavy work load causing MSD			
5	Chances of infection increased			
6	Unsafe play areas or lack of sanitation			
7	Salary is much lower			
8	Job is not permanent			
9	Affects personal life			
10	Less recognition and support			
11	Long working hours			
12	Less staff to help			
13	Loneliness in the work place			

Table 4.2 Factor analysis

	Variable	Factor 1	Factor 2	Factor 3	Factor 4
Occupational risks	1, 2, 11, 12	0.504, 0.519 0.528, 0.559			
Psychological stress	3, 13		0.612, 0.708		
Physical stress	4, 5, 6			0.531, 0.518, 0.636	
Work–life balance	7, 8, 9				0.0603, 0.538, 0.556

Table 4.3 Selected nursery teachers' percentage score

	Questionnaire	Percentage of nursery teachers agreed with the questionnaire
1	Work load is high in educating and for caring	87.45
2	Exhausted emotionally	63.42
3	Challenges in adjusting to the varying behavior of children	65.05
4	Heavy work load causing MSD	59.03
5	Chances of infection increased	43.22
6	Unsafe play areas or lack of sanitation	41.03
7	Salary is much lower	67.20
8	Job is not permanent	61.01
9	Affects personal life	60.01
10	Less recognition and support	70.34
11	Long working hours	68.40
12	Less staff to help	62.12
13	Loneliness in the work place	43.04

PSS scale consists of 10 questions. These ten questions were asked to 420 workers. Table 4.4 shows the PSS scale: 0 = never, 1 = almost never, 2 = sometimes, 3 = fairly often, 4 = very often.

The questionnaire was then circulated among nursery teachers and the PSS score was calculated.

The collected PSS scores are written in reverse order: for 0 we write 4, for 1 we write 3, 2 is always 2, 3 will be 1, and 4 will be 0. It is found that:

- A total score between 0 and 40 means very highly stressed;
- A total score between 0 and 13 means a low level of stress;
- A total score between 14 and 26 means moderate stress;
- A total score between 27 and 40 is high tress.

Table 4.4 PSS scale

PSS question	0	1	2	3	4
How many times in the last month have you felt upset about something that wasn't expected? How many times in the last month have you felt that you couldn't make a difference? Have you noted the noteworthy incidents in your life To what extent have you experienced anxiety and stress in the last month? How often did you feel confident in your ability to handle your personal problems throughout the last month? How frequently did you think that things were going your way in the previous month? How frequently you feel it is un bearable, which done In the past month?					
How many times you are able to bear irritable situation?					
How frequently you have controlled the last month situation?					
How many times situation is beyond control and you are irritated?					
How many times have you found the challenges difficult to handle?					

Table 4.5 PSS scores for teachers (pink-collar employees)

India	36
Bangladesh	30
Nepal	9
Nigeria	24

It is clear from Table 4.5 that Indian teachers are very stressed compared to other countries.

Table 4.5 shows the ranking of nurses country-wise.

4.4 Conclusion

Although they serve a vital role in society, nursery, school, and child-care workers face serious threats to their mental health at work. It takes a mix of professional growth, workplace assistance, and generaladvocacy for better working circumstances to address these dangers. By putting these tactics into practice, we may contribute to ensuring that these essential employees preserve their well-being and job happiness while also being effective in their duties.

References

Čecho, R., Švihrová, V., Čecho, D., Novák, M., and Hudečková, H. (2019). Exposure to mental load and psychosocial risks in kindergarten teachers. *Zdr. Varst.* 58, 120–128. https://doi.org/10.2478/sjph-2019-0016

Faulkner, M., Gerstenblatt, P., Lee, A., Vallejo, V., and Travis, D. (2016). Childcare providers: work stress and personal well-being. *J. Early Child. Res.* 14, 280–293. https://doi.org/10.1177/1476718X14552871

Fináncz, J., Nyitrai, A., Podráczky, J., and Csima, M. (2020). Connections between professional well-being and mental health of early childhood educators. *Int. J. Instr.* 13, 731–746. https://doi.org/10.29333/iji.2020.13445a

Chapter 5
Designing a Framework to Reduce the Mental Work Load and Improve the Mental Health of Workers Engaged in Pink-Collar Jobs

5.1 Introduction

Pink-collar jobs include the jobs of school or nursery teachers, hotel services, nursing and caring services, all which require a lot of physical and mental pressure in handling customers. The customers also vary in gender, age, education, and body type. The level of workers' patience must be high when taking care of these customers, as it involves care-giving. Care-giving, understanding others' feelings, coping with their needs, having low control over the work place, and having limited resources without any help—all this entails emotional hardship, resulting in highly stressful jobs. Both the physical and mental pressure levels are high for pink-collar workers in their work place, so they are not able to balance their work and life and their social or family life. Sometimes they neglect their children, parents, spouse, friends, or relatives and sometimes they neglect themselves. The work pressure and long hours not only create bodily pain in the form of MSDs, but also create mental pressure. Pink-collar workers then suffer depression, stress, anxiety, and so on. Hence in this chapter a framework is suggested for reducing the mental pressure of pink-collar workers using a quality function deployment (QFD) method. Chakraborty and Prasad (2018) used QFD to find and rank cotton fiber properties. Lombardi and Fargnoli (2018) used it for finding hazards in small industry. Satapathy et al. (2013) used it to rank barriers existing in utility service delivery.

5.2 Research Methodology

Pink-collar workers face many challenges in their lives. To reduce their mental stress a study was conducted and suggestions collected from academic experts, nursing, and NGOs. In Table 5.1 (where column 1 = disagree, 2 = totally disagree, 3 = no opinion, 4 = totally agree, 5 = agree) the challenges of pink-collar workers are mentioned and

S. Satapathy et al., *Mental and Occupational Stress Assessment of Pink Collar Workers*, New Perspectives in Behavioral & Health Sciences,
https://doi.org/10.1007/978-981-97-9598-7_5

Table 5.1 Customer requirements/challenges for pink-collar workers

	Question	1	2	3	4	5
1	**Emotional labor**					
2	Low wages and financial insecurity					
3	High workloads and physical strain					
4	Workplace disrespect and stigma					
5	**Stress and mental health issues**					
6	Work–life balance challenges					
7	Lack of recognition and support					

Table 5.2 Requirements for mitigating challenges

	Question	O = 0.2	▲ = 0.4	● = 0.6	◉ = 0.8
1	Creating supportive work place environment				
2	Supporting both emotionally and mentally				
3	Flexible work system in terms of time, shift, and types of job				
4	Ergonomic work place design to reduce strain				
5	Training and professional development work culture				
6	Rewards and recognition by higher management				
7	Work–life balance and taking care of health and well being				
8	Feedback or good grievance in organization				
9	Supportive management and good leadership				

the House of Quality (HOQ) is a matrix-based tool that helps organizations design products that meet customer needs. Table 5.2 Correlation symbols of HOQ are 0.2, 0.4, 0.6, 0.8 etc. are taken for symbols O, ▲, ●, ◉.

Customer requirement data were collected from nurses, hotel services, and nursery school teachers. Overall, 500 data items were collected. Figure 5.1 shows the selected number of workers from health care, hotels, nursery schools, carers, and so on. Most data were collected from nursery school teachers. Figure 5.2 shows the selected pink-collar workers gender-wise. Most female workers were found in nurseries.

5.3 Results and Discussion

Table 5.2 shows suggested hows/requirements for mitigating challenges (see Fig. 5.3 and Table 5.3).

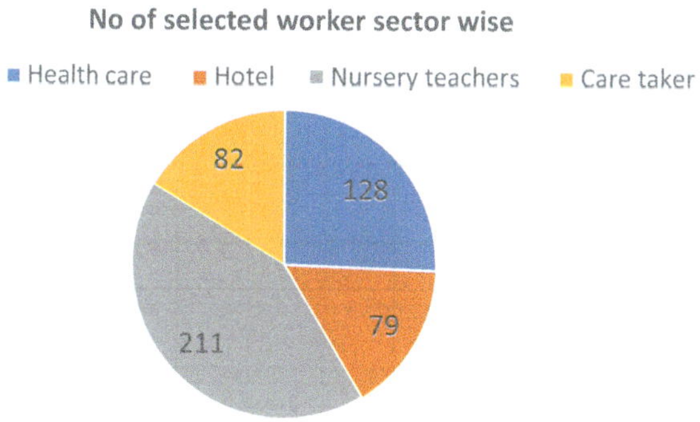

Fig. 5.1 Number of selected workers

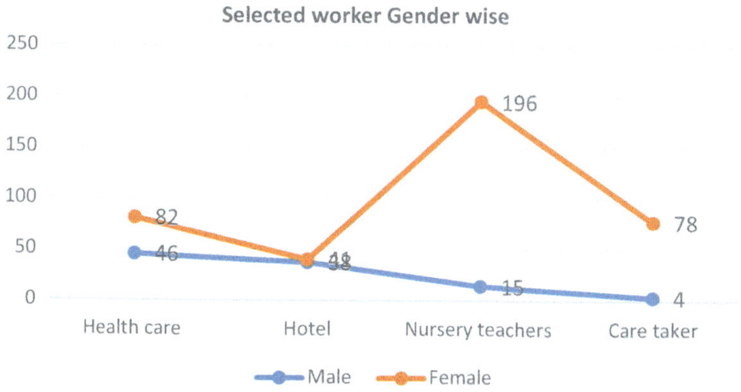

Fig. 5.2 Number of selected workers gender-wise

This framework should be customized to fit the specific needs and circumstances of different workplaces and roles within the pink-collar sector. By addressing both the structural and individual factors that contribute to mental work load and stress, organizations can create healthier, more supportive environments for their workers. By supporting both emotionally and mentally, the mental stress of pink-collar workers can be reduced and ranked first in QFD. With work–life balance and taking care of the health and well being of pink-collar workers may mitigate their mental pressure.

Table 5.3 Designed House of Quality

	requirement	1	2	3	4	5	6	7	8	9	10	Customer rating
1	5	▲	○	•	○	○	•	•	▲		•	2.239
2	1	▲	▲	▲	•	•	•	▲	▲	▲	▲	3.634
3	4	▲	•	•	○	○	•	•	▲		•	4.653
4	1	•	•	▲	•	●	•	▲	▲	▲	○	6.286
5	4	•	▲	▲	▲	○	•	•	▲		•	3.004
6	1	▲	○	•	○	○	•	▲	▲		○	4.119
7	1	•	○	•	▲	○	○	○	○	▲	○	6.490
Initial rating		▲ 8.78	11.28	• 9.054	○ 11.993	7.65	• 7.091	• 13.24	▲ 12.06	8.24	• 10.48	
Revised Rating		11.348	19.48	11.804	14.567	8.28	11.203	18.56	16.78	10.66	12.26	
Normalized Rating		0.582546201	1	0.605954825	0.747792608	0.425051335	0.575102669	0.952772074	0.861396304	0.547227926	0.62936345	
		7th	1st	6th	4th	10th	8th	2nd	3rd	9th	5th	

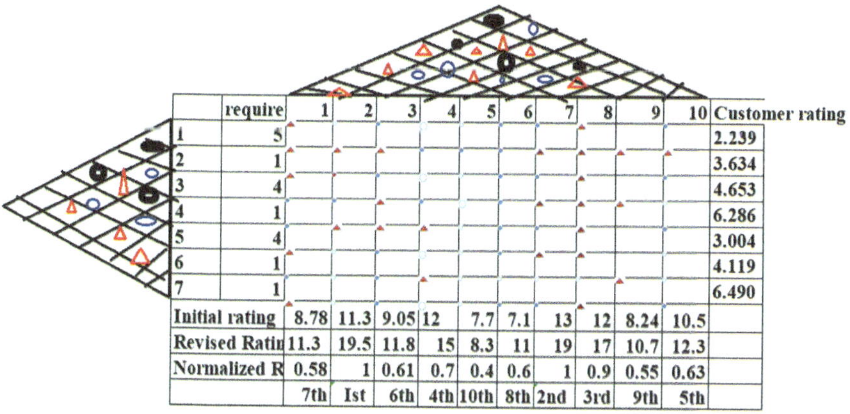

	require	1	2	3	4	5	6	7	8	9	10	Customer rating
1	5											2.239
2	1											3.634
3	4											4.653
4	1											6.286
5	4											3.004
6	1											4.119
7	1											6.490
Initial rating		8.78	11.3	9.05	12	7.7	7.1	13	12	8.24	10.5	
Revised Ratin		11.3	19.5	11.8	15	8.3	11	19	17	10.7	12.3	
Normalized R		0.58	1	0.61	0.7	0.4	0.6	1	0.9	0.55	0.63	
		7th	Ist	6th	4th	10th	8th	2nd	3rd	9th	5th	

Fig. 5.3 House of quality

5.4 Conclusion

Employers, governments, unions, and society at large must work together to mitigate the difficulties experienced by pink-collar workers. A more egalitarian and encouraging work environment for these workers can be achieved by addressing concerns about pay, job security, gender equality, and work–life balance. In addition to enhancing the lives of persons occupying these positions, these initiatives will advance society's general health and well being.

References

Chakraborty, S., & Prasad, K. (2018). A Quality Function Deployment-Based Expert System for Cotton Fibre Selection. *Journal of The Institution of Engineers (India): Series E, 99*(1), 43–53.

Lombardi, M., & Fargnoli, M. (2018). Prioritization of hazards by means of a QFD- based procedure. *International Journal of Safety and Security Engineering, 8*(2), 342–353. https://doi.org/10.2495/SAFE-V8-N2-342-353

Satapathy S, Patel SK, Mahapatra SS, Biswas A. A framework for electricity utility service by QFD technique. International Journal of Services Sciences. 2013 Jan 1;5(1):58–73.

Chapter 6
Exploring the Physical and Mental Pressure of Workers in Hotel Services

6.1 Introduction

The hospitality industry or hotels is both a product and service-based industry, where food quality and hotel service are both important from the customer satisfaction point of view. As it is a very competitive industry, employers and employees experience much pressure and try their best to provide good quality and good hospitality. Work stress varies with types of work. The stress levels of the hotel manager and hotel boys, cooks, security guards, and other service workers are not all the same, like their wages or monthly perks, but altogether their goal is to deliver good service, to attract consumers, and to improve their ratings more than their competitors. With increasing stress levels of employees, work performance decreases and the employer and the business suffer. In this chapter a study is carried out to explore the physical and mental stress of workers in hotel or hospitality services.

Cooper and Payne (1988) discussed work stress among hotel managers. Karasek (1979) proposed a job strain model. Job pressure in the hospitality industry is the main cause of employee reduction according to Cooper and Dewe (2008) and Lazarus (1999). Greenberg and Jin (2005) investigated why workers feel tired when dealing with multifarious clients. Bakar et al. (2015) considered the challenges and stress of the hotels in Asian countries. Igbojekwe (2017) showed the impacts of emotional hardship directly affect the job performance of workers. Rao and Goel (2017) described the factors affecting work-related stress in the hospitality industry. Satapathy (2014) used interpretative structural modeling (ISM) for finding relations in electricity utility services. Satapathy (2024) used ISM for challenges of sustainable supply chain management. Satapathy (2017) found barriers to plastic recycling using an ISM methodology.

S. Satapathy et al., *Mental and Occupational Stress Assessment of Pink Collar Workers*, New Perspectives in Behavioral & Health Sciences,
https://doi.org/10.1007/978-981-97-9598-7_6

6.2 Research Methodology

To study hospitality industry workers' physical and mental pressure, a broad literature review was conducted and based on this and experts' suggestions a standard questionnaire was designed and circulated among the hospitality industries of India, Mexico, Bangladesh, Nepal, Bhutan, and Nigeria. After personal interviews and telephone and mail interaction around 312 data items were collected. Table 6.1 shows the questionnaire, which used the Likert scale (i.e. 1 = totally disagree, 2 = disagree, 3 = no opinion, 4 = agree, and 5 = totally agree). Figure 6.1 shows the selected number of workers country-wise. It was found that the maximum amount of data (130) was collected from India. Table 6.2 shows the types of selected workers based on their work, age, experience, and education.

Table 6.1 Questionnaire

	Work pattern	1	2	3	4	5
1	Long shift work and different patterns of work; irregular hours					
2	Repetitive and heavy physical work load and overtime					
3	Heavy work load and fatigue with MSD risk of accidents and hazards					
4	Work load and time pressure creates anxiety and stress					
5	Insecure job and wage rate is very low, so financially stressed					
6	Due to language barriers, face problems in communicating and understanding					
7	Difficult to handle demanding consumers					
8	Workers have to hide their emotions					

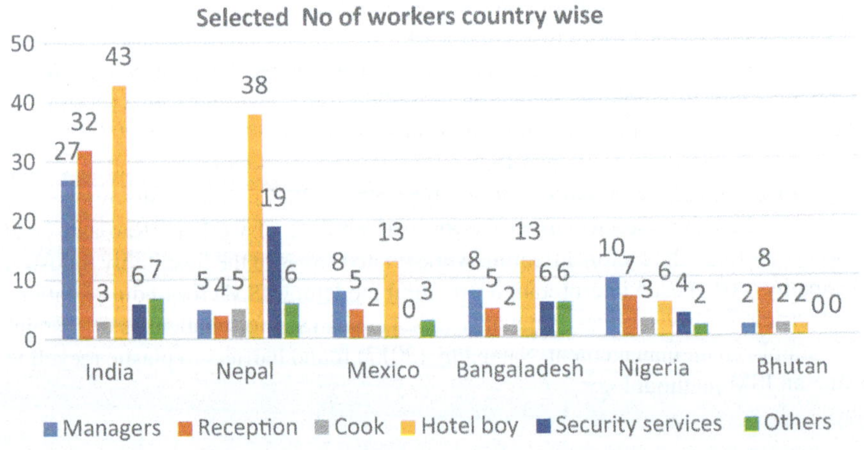

Fig. 6.1 Selected number of workers country-wise

Table 6.2 Types of workers

Workers	No	Experience (years)	Age	Education
Managers	60	5–15	30–55	Masters
Reception	61	5–10	25–35	Graduate
Cook	17	5–10	30–45	12th to graduate
Hotel boy	115	5–10	18–40	12th to graduate
Security services	35	5–15	18–50	12th to graduate
Others	24	5	18–50	School

6.3 Results and Discussion

After collecting the data, Minitab 17 was used to conduct factor analysis and all eight items were selected under two dimensions (i.e. physical pressure and mental pressure). All items had a Cronbach's alpha value of more than 0.5. Table 6.3 shows the factor analysis of the hospitality industry.

ISM was then implemented to find interrelationships between the components or elements of the mental pressure and physical pressure of hospitality workers (see Tables 6.4, 6.5, 6.6, 6.7, 6.8, 6.9, 6.10 and 6.11 and Fig. 6.2).

Figure 6.3 shows MICMAC analysis, with the total variables divided into four clusters. Variable 3 has less dependency; and low drive power is named as the key variable. Variable 4 has low drive power and more dependency falls under group II. Group III variables have more dependency and high drive power. Items 1, 2, 4, 6,

Table 6.3 Factor analysis

	Items	Factor 1	Factor 2
Physical pressure	1, 2, 3	0.811, 0.756, 0.504	
Mental pressure	4, 5, 6, 7, 8		0.639, 0.712, 0.547, 0.563, 0.681

Table 6.4 Self structural interactive matrix

	8	7	6	5	4	3	2	1
1	O	V	V	A	V	O	V	
2	O	V	V	V	V	A		
3	V	O	V	V	V			
4	A	O	V	A				
5	V	O	A					
6	O	A						
7	V							
8								

Table 6.5 Initial reachability matrix

	1	2	3	4	5	6	7	8
1	1	1	0	1	1	1	1	1
2	1	1	0	1	1	1	1	1
3	1	1	1	1	1	1	1	1
4	1	1	0	1	1	1	1	1
5	0	0	0	1	1	1	0	0
6	0	1	0	0	1	1	0	1
7	1	0	0	1	1	1	0	1
8	0	0	0	0	0	0	0	0

Table 6.6 Final reachability matrix with transitivity relationship

	1	2	3	4	5	6	7	8	Driver
1	1	1	0	1	1*	1*	1	1	7
2	1	1	0	1*	1*	1	1	1	7
3	1	1	1	1	1	1	1	1	8
4	1	1	0	1	1	1	1	1	7
5	0	0	0	1	1	1	0	1	4
6	0	1	0	0	1	1	0	1	4
7	1	0	0	1	1*	1	0	1	5
8	1	1*	1	1	0	1	1	1	7
Dependency	7	6	2	7	7	8	5	8	

* shows transitivity relation

Table 6.7 Iteration 1

Variables	Reachability set	Antecedent set	Intersection set	Level
1	1, 2, 4, 5, 6, 7, 8	1, 2, 3, 4, 7, 8	1, 2, 4, 7, 8	
2	1, 2, 4, 5, 6, 7, 8	1, 2, 3, 4, 6.8	1, 2, 4, 6, 8	
3	1, 2, 3, 4, 5, 6, 7, 8	3, 8	3, 8	
4	1, 2, 4, 5, 6, 7, 8	1, 2, 3, 4, 5, 7, 8	1, 2, 4, 5, 7, 8	
5	4, 5, 6, 8	4, 5, 6, 8	4, 5, 6, 8	I
6	2, 5, 6, 8	1, 2, 3, 4, 5, 6, 7	2, 5, 6, 8	I
7	1, 4, 5, 6	1, 2, 3, 4	1, 4	
8	1, 2, 3, 4, 6, 7, 8	1, 2, 3, 4, 5, 6, 7, 8	1, 2, 3, 4, 6, 7, 8	I

Table 6.8 Iteration 2

Variables	Reachability set	Antecedent set	Intersection set	Level
1	1, 2, 4, 7	1, 2, 3, 4, 7	1, 2, 4, 7	II
2	1, 2, 4, 7	1, 2, 3, 4	1, 2, 4	
3	1, 2, 3, 4, 7	3	3	
4	1, 2, 4, 7	1, 2, 3, 4, 7	1, 2, 4, 7	II
7	1, 4	1, 2, 3, 4	1, 4	II

Table 6.9 Iteration 3

Variables	Reachability set	Antecedent set	Intersection set	Level
2	2	2, 3	2	III
3	2, 3	3	3	

Table 6.10 Iteration 4

Variables	Reachability set	Antecedent set	Intersection set	Level
3	3	3	3	IV

Table 6.11 MIC MAC analysis

									Driver
8									7
7		IV			7	III	1, 5	8	7
6								6	8
5						2			7
4		3					4		4
3		I					II		4
2									5
1									7
Dependency	7	6	2	7	7	8	5	8	
	1	2	3	4	5	6	7	8	

and 8 come under this category. Group IV variables have more drive power and less dependency. No variable falls into this group.

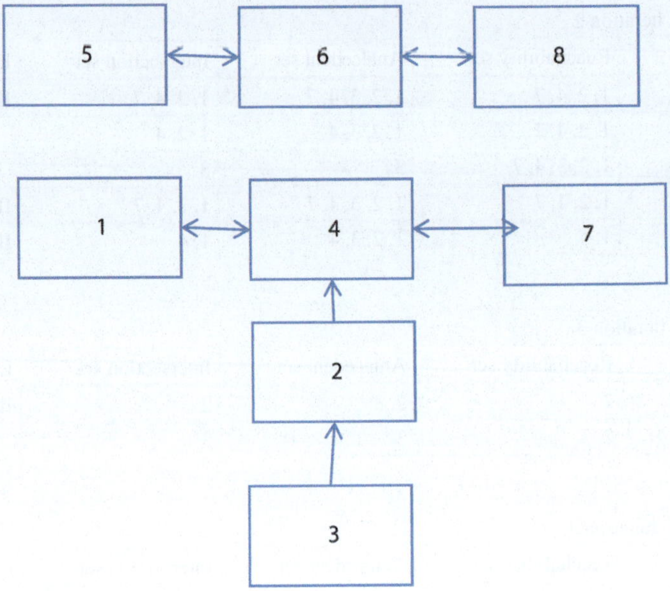

Fig. 6.2 ISM model

									Driver
8									7
7		IV			7	III	1,5	8	7
6								6	8
5						2			7
4		3					4		4
3		I					II		4
2									5
1									7
Dependency	7	6	2	7	7	8	5	8	
	1	2	3	4	5	6	7	8	

Fig. 6.3 MICMAC analysis

6.4 Conclusion

The hospitality sector is renowned for its high standards and fast-paced work environment, which may put employees under a lot of physical and psychological strain. Here is a look at both of them. The substantial physical and psychological strains that hotel employees endure may have a negative impact on their health and general well-being. Resolving these issues calls for an all-encompassing strategy that incorporates enhancing working conditions, offering sufficient assistance, and encouraging a respectful and considerate work environment.

References

Bakar KA, Salleh AM, Muda MS, Ahmad A, Manshor R. Challenge-stress and hindrance-stress in the Southeast Asian hotel sector. Journal of Indonesian Economy and Business: JIEB.. 2015 May 1;30(2):101.

Cooper G, Green JC, Payne MP. Relative partial photoionization cross-sections and photoelectron branching ratios of the valence-bands of the group VIII metallocenes of iron, ruthenium and osmium. Molecular Physics. 1988 Apr 20;63(6):1031–51.

Cooper C, Dewe PJ. Stress: A brief history. John Wiley & Sons; 2008 Apr 15.

Greenberg DA, Jin K. From angiogenesis to neuropathology. Nature. 2005 Dec 15;438(7070):954–9.

Igbojekwe P. Impacts of Emotional Labour on Employee Job Performance in Hotels in South East Nigeria. International Journal of Applied Research. 2017;3(7):943–53.

Karasek Jr RA. Job demands, job decision latitude, and mental strain: Implications for job redesign. Administrative science quarterly. 1979 Jun 1:285–308.

Lazarus RS (1999) Stress and Emotion: A New Synthesis. New York: Springer.

Rao E, Goel A. Factors causing work related stress in the Hospitality Sector: A study of employees in three star hotels in Dehradun Region. IARS' International Research Journal. 2017 Feb 8;7(1).

Satapathy S. ANN, QFD and ISM approach for framing electricity utility service in India for consumer satisfaction. International Journal of Services and Operations Management. 2014 Jan 1;18(4):404–28.

Satapathy S. An analysis of barriers for plastic recycling in the Indian plastic industry. Benchmarking: An International Journal. 2017 Mar 6;24(2):415–30.

Satapathy S. Sustainable Supply Chain Management Challenges in Petroleum Transportation: As per Indian Perspective. In Strategies for Environmentally Responsible Supply Chain and Production Management 2024 (pp. 182–205). IGI Global.

Chapter 7
Conclusion and Study of the Changing Scenario of the Pink-Collar-Worker Industry

7.1 Introduction

Pink-collar jobs are care-oriented jobs, usually considered as female jobs. The beauty industries, social work, teaching jobs, secretarial jobs, and so on are included within pink-collar jobs. This workers' scenario has changed. Many male employees are also taking part in pink-collar jobs nowadays, but in comparison to females they are still less in number. They work in particular in hospitals to handle male patients, to check their health, or to take care of them. This has resolved many problems of female nurses working in hospitals.

To handle infants in child care services requires a lot of patience and physical and mental labor. Men cannot handle such situations well and the requirement for females is greater. For nursery teachers, being naturally motherly, female workers can teach and groom children with the required proper care. So here too female workers are required.

Similarly in the hospitality industry, although the ratio of males to females is less, it is not zero. From the manager to the hotel boy, diverse roles are needed for the satisfaction of clients, which female workers can perform with patience. Hence female workers are required here.

As secretary, clerk, or beautician, female workers labor in diverse fields, with the requisite patience, also leading to more female employees than male ones.

7.2 Study of the Changing Scenario of the Pink-Collar Industry

Pink-collar workers' places of employment and industrial scenario have changed. Hard manual labor has changed and become automated, making life comfortable and easy. The game changers of pink-collar workers' lives are:

S. Satapathy et al., *Mental and Occupational Stress Assessment of Pink Collar Workers*, New Perspectives in Behavioral & Health Sciences,
https://doi.org/10.1007/978-981-97-9598-7_7

1. Advanced technology: Due to AI and advanced technology, much work is automated. Hence heavy physical work, repetitive work, and so on has changed. To adopt new technology training and learn skills are very essential. Digital scheduling tools help workers to schedule work loads and communicate properly. Tele-health platforms also help in proper customer interaction. With the help of customer service management software/apps the difficult jobs of hotels are streamlined, reducing overburdening by tasks. Digital teaching processes, computer games, educational play, and teaching software also help to engage small children by reducing the stress of nursery teachers.
2. Virtual platforms due to the pandemic: After the pandemic pink-collar workers, particularly in the health care sector, have received more recognition, due to their dedicated service. This has also impacted their wage rate and socioeconomic respect. Hybrid modes of teaching, retailing, and administrative responsibilities are now feasible for some pink-collar workers, making their work and work-life balance better.
3. **Workforce demographic changes**: The pink-collar workforce was previously female based, but nowadays it is more diverse in nature. The entry of men in conventional female-dominated roles like child care, taking care of seniors, and cooking has shown that pink-collar workers' jobs are also professional in nature. This diversity has given recognition and social respect and value to these workers.
4. **Development of law, policy, and standard regulation**: The pink-collar job now has professional recognition and the scale and fixed pay/wage rate has increased. By observing the essential of job certain rules, do's and don'ts have implemented for pink-collar workers. Like other workers with structured packages, medical benefits, house rent, and leave rules have been implemented, which makes these jobs more secure.
5. To take care of **mental health and well-being**: To take care of pink-collar workers, employers are giving priority to their mental health. For this, certain mental wellness, stress management, and resilience training programs are introduced. Even work place flexibility is provided for these workers by introducing part-time work, job sharing, and flexible scheduling. This will help to make a balance between family and work life.

7.3 Methodology

Pink-collar workers are those who work in occupations that are normally associated with women, such as nursing, teaching, providing care, and administrative positions. The phrase itself alludes to the gendered character of these fields, which have traditionally been dominated by women. The landscape for workers in the pink-collar sector has been changing as a result of numerous socioeconomic developments, advances in technology, and changes in public perception. Here are some thoughts and viewpoints from workers in the pink-collar industry in this evolving environment. Table 7.1 shows the responses in yes and no format.

Table 7.1 Opinions on the changes in the pink-collar industry

	Opinions	Yes = 1	No = 0
1	Recognition has increased		
2	No development in financial conditions		
3	Job security is questionable due to automation		
4	Technology has made possible flexibility and remote working		
5	Due to its being gender-specific work, it is undervalued		
6	Entry of men may help in increasing wage and recognition		
7	There is an increasing push for unionization and collective bargaining		
8	Policies for paternal leave are being made		
9	Economic inequality		

Fifty pink-collar workers with experience of working in the changing scenario were then asked to give their opinion. Statistical analysis, linear regression analysis, and the TOPSIS MCDM method was then performed on the collected data.

7.4 Results and Discussion

After analyzing the collected data, it was found (see Table 7.2) that 86% of pink-collar workers agree that recognition of their profession has increased.

When the resopnses of pink collar workers are considered as independent variable and predicted against Well ness of pink collar workers, Well ness of pink collar workers is considered as dependent variable. Regression model is represented in Fig. 7.1 a residual plot which is generated showing predicted value and fitness of the regression model. It shows an R-squared value of 0.713, which means this model displays the best fitness factor.

Table 7.2 Pink-collar workers who report a positive response (%)

	Opinions	
1	Recognition has increased	86
2	No development in financial conditions	26
3	Job security is questionable due to automation	28
4	Technology has made possible flexibility and remote working	76
5	Due to its being gender-specific work, it is undervalued	6.5
6	Entry of men may help in increasing wage and recognition	24
7	There is an increasing push for unionization and collective bargaining	12
8	Policies for paternal leave are being made	66.6
9	Economic inequality	36

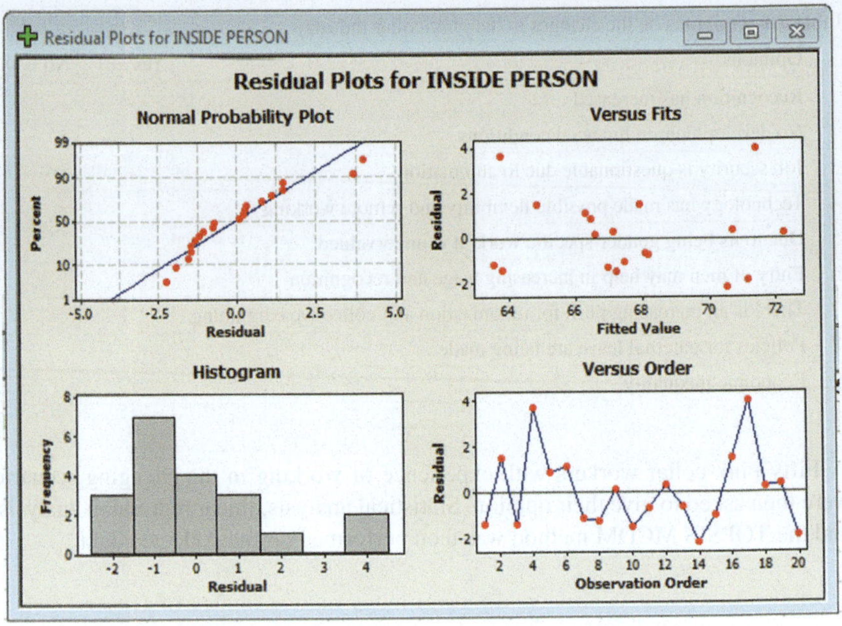

Fig. 7.1 Residual plot

A linear regression model was implemented by using Minitab software.

Y = Wellness of pink-collar workers.

X1, X2, X3, X4, X5, X6, X7, X8, X9 are dependent variables, including requested opinions.

Y = 48.7 + 1.92 X1 − 1.90 X2 − 0.37 X3 + 0.083 X4 + 0.215 X5 − 0.088 X6 + 0.28 X7 − 0.008 X8 + 0.64 X9.

The TOPSIS method was used to rank or prioritize the workers regarding their work place. Tables 7.3, 7.4, 7.5, 7.6, 7.7 and 7.8 are the steps of the TOPSIS MCDM method used.

For the TOPSIS method, a range is taken from 1 to 5 (i.e. worst, Bad, normal, good, excellent).

From the ranking shown in Table 7.8, it is seen that A3 (healthcare) workers have benefited most due to changes in the work place due to advanced technology, followed by nursery teachers ranked second and hotel workers ranked third.

Table 7.3 Criteria for pink-collar workers

Criteria	
Recognition has increased	P1
No development in financial conditions	P2
Job security is questionable due to automation	P3
Technology has made possible flexibility and remote working	P4
Due its being gender-specific work, it is undervalued	P5
Entry of men may help in increasing wage and recognition	P6
There is an increasing push for unionization and collective bargaining	P7
Policies for paternal leave are being made	P8
Economic inequality	P9

Table 7.4 Alternatives

Nursery school teacher job	A1
Hospitality job	A2
Healthcare work	A3
Clerical job	A4

Table 7.5 Decision matrix criteria

Alternatives	P1	P2	P3	P4	P5	P6	P7	P8	P9
A1	5	4	4	4	3	5	4	3	2
A2	3	2	3	4	5	4	2	5	4
A3	5	4	3	2	4	4	4	3	4
A4	5	4	3	5	5	2	4	3	4
$\sqrt{\sum^{M} Xij^2}$ $I = 1$	9.165	7.211	6.557	7.810	8.660	7.810	7.211	7.211	7.211

Table 7.6 Normalized values

Weighing	0.25	0.25	0.25	0.25	0.25	0.25	0.25	0.25	0.25
	P1	P2	P3	P4	P5	P6	P7	P8	P9
A1	0.327	0.5547	0.4575	0.5121	0.5774	0.5121	0.5547	0.4160	0.5547
A2	0.5355	0.5547	0.4575	0.5121	0.5774	0.6402	0.5547	0.6934	0.5547
A3	0.5458	0.5547	0.6100	0.6402	0.4619	0.5121	0.5547	0.4160	0.5547
A4	0.535	0.2774	0.4575	0.2561	0.3464	0.2561	0.2774	0.4160	0.2774

Table 7.7 Positive and negative ideal solutions

Alternatives	Si+	Si–	Si+ + Si–	Ci
A1	0.3696	0.4487	0.8183	0.548321
A2	0.3903	0.3906	0.7809	0.500153
A3	0.3227	0.3972	0.7199	0.551751
A4	0.3537	0.2908	0.6445	0.451164

Table 7.8 Ranking

Alternatives	Ci	Rank
A1	0.548321	2
A2	0.500153	3
A3	0.551751	1
A4	0.451164	4

7.4.1 Conclusion and Future Scope

To create a sustainable work force, pink-collar workers' physical and mental health must be good. They must be able to live happily with prosperity like others in society. They need to be respected in society as their jobs are highly emotionally demanding. Pink-collar work is about to undergo a huge shift. The sector may come to experience better working conditions, higher pay, and more prospects for professional advancement as society comes to value it more. It will be essential to make investments in workers' professional growth, well-being, and working environment in order to create a more sustainable and equitable workforce. Understanding how to best help these workers in this evolving scenario will require ongoing research and trend tracking.

Index

A
Allowance, 3, 16
Automation, 41, 42

B
Blue collar, 5, 11
Business, 31

C
Challenges, 3, 11, 12, 20–22, 25, 26, 31
Child care, 1, 19, 20, 39, 40
Climate-changes, 6
Community, 2

D
Design, 26

E
Ergonomic, 3, 6, 26

F
Female, 2, 3, 6, 11, 16, 26, 39, 40

G
Gender, 3, 6, 16, 25–27, 29, 41, 42

H
Health, 1–3, 5–7, 11, 16, 19, 23, 26, 28, 29, 37, 39, 40, 44
Hospital, 3, 6, 14, 15, 39
Hospitality, 3, 6, 31–33, 37, 39
Hotel, 1, 5, 25, 26, 31, 33, 37, 39, 40, 44

I
Industry, 1, 25, 31–33, 39–41
Innovative, 6

M
Measurement, 2, 6, 20
Men, 11, 39–42
Mental stress, 3, 11, 19, 20, 31
Mental workload, 13, 14
Multi-Criteria Decision-Making (MCDM), 12, 13, 41, 42
Musculoskeletal disorders, 1, 16

N
Nurse, 6, 11–13, 16, 23, 26, 39
Nursery, 1, 5, 19–21, 23, 25, 26, 39, 40, 43, 44

O
Organisation, 7, 26, 28

P
Physical, 1–3, 6, 11, 13, 19–21, 25, 26, 31–33, 37, 39, 40, 44
Pink collar, 1
Policy, 16, 40

S. Satapathy et al., *Mental and Occupational Stress Assessment of Pink Collar Workers*, New Perspectives in Behavioral & Health Sciences,
https://doi.org/10.1007/978-981-97-9598-7

Prediction, 41
Productivity, 2, 16
Pshychological, 21

Q
Quality, 2, 25–28, 31
Question, 12, 16, 20–22, 26, 32

R
Reduction, 3, 31

S
Safety, 2, 5, 6
Sickness, 16
Strain, 11, 26, 31, 37
Stress, 2, 6, 7, 13, 16, 19–22, 25, 26, 28, 31, 32, 40
Sustainable, 6, 31, 44

T
Threat, 23

W
Well being, 19, 20, 26, 28, 29
Wellness, 19, 40, 41
Women, 1, 3, 6, 11, 40
Workload, 13, 14, 26

The manufacturer's authorised representative in the EU is Springer Nature Customer Service Centre GmbH, Europaplatz 3, 69115 Heidelberg, Germany. If you have any concerns regarding our products, please contact ProductSafety@springernature.com

Printed and bound by CPI Group (UK) Ltd, Croydon, CR0 4YY

01/10/2026

02225880-0001